Al Mahady Toure
Patrick Thonneau
Modibo Keïta

Efficacy´ of trichiasis surgery and degree´ of satisfaction.

Al Mahady Toure
Patrick Thonneau
Modibo Keïta

Efficacy of trichiasis surgery and degree of satisfaction.

Trichiasis: an added burden

ScienciaScripts

Imprint
Any brand names and product names mentioned in this book are subject to trademark, brand or patent protection and are trademarks or registered trademarks of their respective holders. The use of brand names, product names, common names, trade names, product descriptions etc. even without a particular marking in this work is in no way to be construed to mean that such names may be regarded as unrestricted in respect of trademark and brand protection legislation and could thus be used by anyone.

Cover image: www.ingimage.com

This book is a translation from the original published under ISBN 978-620-6-72332-5.

Publisher:
Sciencia Scripts
is a trademark of
Dodo Books Indian Ocean Ltd. and OmniScriptum S.R.L publishing group

120 High Road, East Finchley, London, N2 9ED, United Kingdom
Str. Armeneasca 28/1, office 1, Chisinau MD-2012, Republic of Moldova, Europe
Printed at: see last page
ISBN: 978-620-8-33008-8

Acknowledgements :

To the entire administration of Senghor University, as well as to the teaching staff, please find in this work the expression of our most sincere thanks for the efforts you have made to provide us with quality training.

To our former Department Director, **Dr François Marie LAHAYE**; To you, **Dr Patrick THONNEAU**, our Department Director;

To you, **Mrs Alice**, Head of the department's administrative service; I cannot express enough my great gratitude for your availability, your support, your advice and the quality of your supervision in the preparation of this work.

To **Professor Lamine TRAORE**, Coordinator of the national eye health program and supervisor; I would like to thank you for the time and interest you devoted to us despite your commitments and responsibilities, as well as all the staff made available to us for the survey (**Mr Sidiki TOGOLA, Mahamadou. DOUMBIA, Mr. Abdramane BENGALY, Mr. COULIBALY Famolo**).

We would like to express our sincere thanks to **Ms Marely KENIERMEN**, former Director of HKI Mali, for having accepted us into the organization and provided us with all the necessary means to carry out this study. **Mohamed L. YATTARA**; **Dr Benoît DEMBELE**, MTN program coordinator at HKI Mali; **Dr Modibo KEITA**, co-supervisor and coordinator of the trachoma project at HKI Mali); **Dr Seydou Goïta**, coordinator of the Lymphatic Filariasis project at HKI Mali; **Dr Fama KONDO, assistant chief of staff at HKI Mali**. **Fama KONDO**, Assistant Project Manager at HKI Mali; **Dr Mama DOUMBIA**, Assistant Project Manager at HKI Mali); **Dr Boubacar GUINDO**, MTN Program Monitoring and Evaluation Officer at HKI Mali; the Hilton Project Regional Coordinator, **Mr Dramane TRAORE** and all the staff at HKI Mali for their daily support. This work is yours. To the chief physicians, the heads of the ophthalmology department and all the staff of the Kita and Diéma health districts who made themselves available to us for their contributions and support during the completion ofthis work, please accept the expression of our deepest gratitude.

We would like to express our gratitude to our promotion colleagues for their contribution.

Health International

Signing sessions

I dedicate this work to: my two parents: the late **AL Kalifa and Haoua Idrissa TOURE**; thanks to God and to you, I am here.

To my wife, **Fatimata KARABENTA**; may the good Lord shower you with his grace for all your sacrifice, patience and support, and may he bless our home.

My children, may this work influence your creativity to always do better, and serve as a reference point for serving humanity in health, prosperity and, above all, peace. self-sacrifice.

To my uncle Moussa Idrissa TOURE for his unfailing blessings.

My sisters (Anna, Hadeye, Hamsa, Fatto, Maimouna, Badji) and their husbands especially to **Abdoulaye M'BAYE** for your support; and brothers (Djibril, Sékou, Sabane, Alhousseyni, Alassane), our late father is proud of us because you had my back as always, showing that family unity is sacred. Thanks to you, I haven't had to worry about a thing for the past two years. This work is yours.

Summary:

Introduction: According to the World Health Organization, trachomatous trichiasis (TT) is the leading preventable cause of infectious blindness worldwide. It is the final stage in the evolution of trachoma before blindness. Badly operated, trichiasis can recur and continue its progression towards irreversible blindness, making families even more precarious.

Objective: Our study aimed to assess the quality of TT surgery and patient satisfaction in the Kayes region of Mali.

Methodology: This was a cross-sectional study conducted from June 22 to July 1er 2018 among 125 people randomly selected from the 492 people operated on for trichiasis in 2017 in the Kita and Diema health districts, one year after the operation. An experienced ophthalmologist examined the eyes using a magnifying glass with 2.5 dioptres magnification and a lamp, to detect any recurrences and complications recorded in a standard questionnaire. Eye care was provided, where necessary, with the participant's informed consent.

Results: Women accounted for 62% (77/125) of participants, with a majority over 60 years of age (66%, 82/125) and a median age of 65 years, with a minimum of 31 years and a maximum of 101 years. The study revealed 14.9% (25/167) recurrences at one year after surgery, with a high frequency in women (72%, 18/25). Cases of granuloma-type complications were not numerous 2% (3/125). The study also reported that among TT surgery recipients 66% (83/125) received Azithromicin immediately after surgery. Among those who underwent surgery, 95% (119/125) were satisfied with the outcome of their operation, compared with just 2% (2/125) who were not at all satisfied and 3% (4/125) who had no opinion.

Conclusion: Our study shows that TT surgery in these two districts is of acceptable quality. Indeed, TT surgery is a priority in the elimination of trachoma. In Mali, the National Eye Health Program and its partners, including Helen Keller International, have been working towards this goal since 2007. Given that studies have shown that there can be no such thing as an absence of recurrence, preventing and/or reducing the occurrence of complications would guarantee the success of any program

.**Key words:** Surgery, Trichiasis, Quality, satisfaction, Mali

Abstract:

Introduction: According to the World Health Organization, trachomatous trichiasis (TT) is the leading preventable cause of blindness of infectious origin in the world. It is the ultimate stage in the evolution of trachoma before blindness. Poorly operated, trichiasis can recur and continue its evolution towards irreversible blindness, thus aggravating the precariousness of families.

Objective: Our study aimed to assess the quality of TT surgery and patient satisfaction in the Kayes region of Mali.

Methodology: This was a cross-sectional study conducted from 22 June to 1 July 2018 with 125 people randomly selected from among the 492 people operated for trichiasis in 2017 in the Kita and Diema health districts one year after the intervention. An experienced ophthalmologist examines the eyes with a 2.5 diopter magnification magnifying glass and a lamp to detect possible recurrences and complications recorded in a standard questionnaire. Eye care was provided, where applicable, with the informed consent of the participant.

Results: Women constituted 62% (77/125) of participants with a majority over 60 years of age 66% (82/125) and a median age of 65 years with a minimum of 31 years and a maximum of 101 years. In the study, 15% (25/167) of recurrences occurred at one year after surgery with a high frequency in women 72% (18/25) of recurrences. Cases of granuloma-type complications were not numerous at 2% (3/125). The study also reported that among TT surgery beneficiaries 66% (83/125) received Azithromicin immediately after surgery. Among surgical beneficiaries 95% (119 /125) were satisfied with the outcome of their operation compared to only 2% (2 /125) who were not at all satisfied and 3% (4 /125) who were without opinion.

Conclusion: Our study shows that TT surgery in these two districts is of acceptable quality. Indeed, TT surgery is a priority axis in the elimination of trachoma. In Mali, the National Eye Health Program with its partners, including Helen Keller International, has been working since 2007 to achieve this objective. Since studies have shown that there can be no recurrence, preventing and/or reducing the occurrence of complications would be a key to the success of any program.

Keywords: Surgery, Trichiasis, Quality, satisfaction, Mali

List of acronyms and abbreviations :

AMO: Ophthalmic Medical Assistant

CHANCE: Trichiasis surgery, Antibiotic therapy to treat Chlamydia trachomatis infection, Facial cleansing and Environmental change.

CSRef: Centre de santé de référence

HKI: Helen Keller International

ODK: Open data kit

WHO: World Health Organization **NGO**: Non-Governmental Organization **OPT:** Operateur du Trichiasis

PCT: Trachoma Control Program **PNSO:** National Eye Health Program **TSO:** Technicien Supérieur en Ophtalmologie **TT:** Trachomatous Trichiasis

Contents:

Introduction :

Described by the Egyptians over 3,500 years ago, trachoma is one of the oldest known diseases[1] . Present on every continent in the first half of the last century, it has completely disappeared from industrialized countries thanks to the improvement in socio-economic and health conditions in these countries[1] . A neglected tropical disease, trachoma is the leading infectious cause of blindness worldwide[2–4] . It is caused by the micro-organism *Chlamydia trachomatis*, which is transmitted by contact with the ocular secretions (via towels, handkerchiefs, fingers and flies) of the infected person[5] . Modern medicine has established the link between repeated childhood infections with Chlamydia trachomatis and adult trichiasis[6] . After years of repeated reinfections, the inside of the eyelid scleroses and turns inwards (entropion), with the eyelashes rubbing against the eyeball (trichiasis), particularly the cornea. Trachomatous trichiasis is extremely painful[7] . If left untreated, entropion- trichiasis can lead to corneal opacities and irreversible blindness .[8]

Blinding trachoma is only endemic in areas where access to water is difficult, overcrowding and poor personal and community hygiene (due to a lack of latrines and sanitation facilities); living with an infected person and poverty in general are also risk factors .[9]

The consequences of active trachoma appear in adults. They often strike the most vulnerable members of communities, women and children. In hyper-endemic areas, active disease is most common in pre-school children, with prevalences reaching 60-90%[8] . Adult women are at far greater risk of developing the blinding complications of the disease than men .[8]

Trachoma is an obstacle to development because of the disability and dependence it causes in infected individuals. The infection often begins in early childhood and can become chronic[10] . Trachomatous trichiasis is responsible for visual impairment and blindness in 1.9 million people, or around 1.4% of total blindness cases worldwide. Timely surgery for trichiasis can prevent a large number of cases of blindness .[8]

Trachoma is a public health problem in 26 countries in the World Health Organization

(WHO) African region. In 2016, of the 260,000 cases of trichiasis more than 247,000 were operated on in this region, representing 95% of all procedures worldwide .[8]

The burden of trachoma on affected individuals and communities is considerable. Its economic cost in terms of lost productivity due to visual impairment and blindness, is estimated at between 2.9 and 5.3 billion dollars (US) per year, 8 billion when trichiasis is included .[11]

In Mali, surveys carried out since the 1980s have shown that the prevalence of trachomatous disease is high in many regions, often exceeding the 25% threshold[12] . The first nationwide mapping carried out between 1996 and 1997 showed a very high prevalence of 34.9% of follicular trachoma (FT) in children aged 1 to 9. The Kayes region was one of the worst affected, with a TF prevalence of 42.5% in children aged 1 to 9, and trachomatous trichiasis (TT) of 3.3% in the population. This mapping was on a regional scale, not a health district scale .[13]

In 1997, WHO created the Alliance for Global Elimination of Trachoma by the Year 2020 (GET2020) .[14]

To eliminate trachoma as a public health problem, a country must have, in each district, a prevalence of trachomatous trichiasis of less than 0.2% of adults aged over 15 (i.e. around 1 case per 1,000 inhabitants) and a prevalence of follicular trachomatous inflammation of less than 5% in children aged 1 to 9. Beyond these prevalences, the WHO recommends the CHANCE strategy to its member countries: surgery to correct trichiasis, antibiotics to treat the infection, for which azithromicin is recommended, facial cleansing and environmental change to interrupt transmission .[5]

Since 1998, the Programme National de Lutte contre la Cécité (PNLC), now Mali's Programme National de Santé Oculaire (PNSO), has been organizing trichiasis surgery days (quinzaines) at least once a year in endemic districts. The free service was introduced in 2005, thanks to the support of technical and financial partners who granted subsidies to Mali to help it achieve its goal of eliminating trachoma .[13]

Since 2007, Helen Keller International (HKI), in collaboration with the PNSO, has been supporting the Kayes region in the fight against trachoma. Trichiasis surgery was selected as a priority activity in this strategy, with teams consisting of an Ophthalmic Medical Assistant (AMO) or a Trichiasis Operator (OPT).

While national eye health programs are moving towards the elimination of trachoma by intensifying surgical treatment and training health professionals in TT surgery, questions are being raised about the quality of these surgeries. Numerous studies have suggested that the recurrence of trichiasis after surgery is partly related to surgical skill or performance[15] . A study of trichiasis surgery patients in The Gambia found that one-year recurrence rates varied between surgeons (from 0% to 83%)[16] . In Tanzania, recurrence rates varied according to district, ranging from 16% to 38% where surgery was performed .[17]

At the first world scientific meeting on trachoma in 2012 in Moshi, Tanzania, and following a study drawn up by the Kilimanjaro Center for Community Ophthalmology, the Carter Center and HKI, recommendations were made on improving the quality of trichiasis surgery[18] . While the number of cases operated on was insufficient, little attention was paid to quality, especially as regards failure in the post-operative period from three to six (3-6) months or even a year .[19]

The recognition of trichiasis as a stage of trachoma, and its distinction from pseudotrichiasis, prompted physicians in earlier times to use a large number of pharmaceutical and surgical treatments[20] . However, not only was the number of cases operated on insufficient, but also the quality of the treatment received little attention .[19]

The usual measure of the quality of TT surgery is the proportion of operated eyes showing recurrence, ranging from 10% after one year to 60% after three years[21] . Two categories are distinguished: early recurrence (0-3 months) due to surgical factors and late recurrence due to progressive scar disease.

Previous studies have reported very frequent cases of recurrence[16,17,22,23] . Various factors such as variations in the relative severity of preoperative TT, continued exposure to *C. trachomatis* infection, quality of surgical training, volume of surgery performed, surgical technique and suture material may influence long-term outcomes .[17]

As surgeon training is of variable quality and not always adequately supervised, it can lead to an increase in cases of recurrence of TT after surgery. It has been shown that surgeons who perform only a few trichiasis procedures per month also tend to have poor results, leading to a vicious circle: few patients, low productivity, poor quality of the procedure and derisory results .[24]

Another study, carried out under operational conditions, reported significant variability in recurrence rates between surgeons (0-80%)[16] . It is therefore not easy to find a reference level for a universally "acceptable" recurrence rate, or to suggest categorized benchmarks based on a combination of these factors.

Once trichiasis has set in, surgery is the only way to prevent visual impairment and blindness .[25]

Conceptual framework:

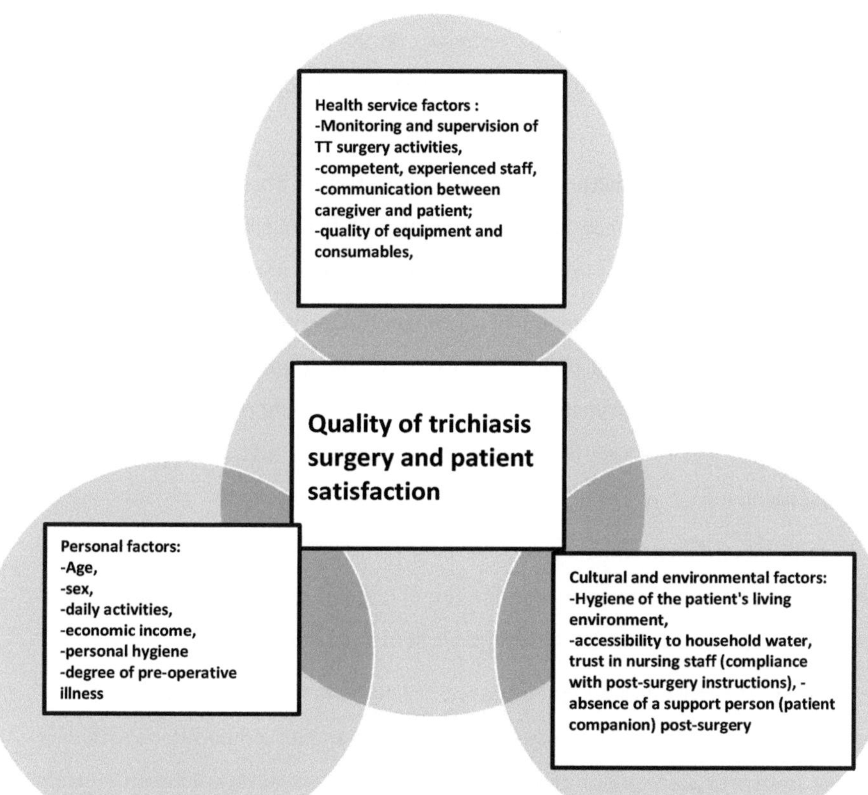

Figure 1: Conceptual framework for trachomatous trichiasis .[16,21–23]

Description of the conceptual framework

Factors that contribute to the failure or impact on the quality of trichiasis surgery can be grouped into three categories: health service factors, cultural and environmental factors, and patient factors.

- **Factors linked to health services:** these are factors observed and/or reported within the health system that can have an impact on the quality of trichiasis surgery. These include factors such as insufficient follow-up mechanisms for TT cases,

weaknesses in the implementation of TT surgery activities, inadequate supervision during the campaign period. Other factors contributing to the poor quality of TT surgery are the number of years of experience, the low number of patients operated on per month, and the lack of mastery of the technique and competence through ongoing training .[17]

- **Cultural and environmental factors**: poor community hygiene, difficult access to clean running water, absence and/or non-use of latrines, difficult access to health care and services, prioritization of traditional treatment and family influence.

- **Personal factors:** In addition to age and sex, these factors refer to personal conditions that predispose to the onset of the disease and its complications, including the occurrence of post-surgical recurrence of trichiasis. Poverty (low economic income) is one of the factors favoring the onset of trachoma itself, non-compliance with post-surgery instructions, late recourse to treatment, poor personal hygiene, not forgetting human biology, which is a determining factor in health. All the factors listed above can influence the quality of TT surgery .[17]

The question of the acceptability of trichiasis surgery is difficult to answer. It takes into account the existence and frequency of relapses at a distance from the operation, the status of operators who are more or less respected by the population, and the financial cost of the operation. It is also difficult to place trichiasis surgery in the context of other eye procedures. It should also be noted that trichiasis surgery has no miraculous effect on the onset of cataracts. Finally, there are some trichiasis operations from which the patient can nevertheless derive a certain degree of comfort, even if the blindness is too advanced to be incurable (depending on how advanced the disease was before surgery). All these circumstances contribute to blurring the image of surgery and its impact, and do not encourage people to adhere to a program whose contours are unclear in terms of immediate and, above all, long-term benefits .[6]

Thus, from the mobile teams approach with outings by motorcycle and car and that of fixed centers, it is the "door-to-door" strategy that is being implemented to reduce the[a] backlog of trichiasis to be operated on, in order to achieve the target set at less than 10% recurrences[18] . These surgical activities are carried out at household level by AMOs, Eye Health Technicians (TSOs) and OPTs in the health districts, with support from the regional and/or national level through ophthalmologists and other experts in the field. This is one of the reasons why relapse after surgery is a considerable obstacle to greater acceptance of TT surgery by the patient .[26]

As each program should determine its own benchmark for the maximum acceptable recurrence rate[31] , more research is needed to improve surgical outcomes for TT patients at high risk of blindness and recurrent trichiasis.In the absence of published data on this subject in Mali, we conducted this study to assess the quality of surgery (recurrence, frequency of complications) and the degree of satisfaction of patients operated on for trachomatous trichiasis in the Kayes region.

.

[1] The number of trichiasis cases awaiting surgery in Mali, approximately 7051 in 2016 Programme National de Santé Oculaire Mali

Methodology :

1.1. Study framework:

Located in the heart of West Africa, Mali is a continental country. The climate is tropical, with alternating dry and rainy seasons lasting an average of 5 months in the south and less than 3 months in the north, and very wide temperature variations.

The hydraulic network is made up of two major rivers, the Niger and the Senegal, serving mainly the south and west of the country and part of the north.

In 2018, this population was estimated at around 18 million, with a poverty rate of 47.1%, a gender inequality index of 0.689 and a human development index of 0.419[27] . The population growth rate was 3.6%. The majority of the country's population lives in rural areas (74.5%). Spatial distribution is uneven. At the last census, only 22.5% of the resident population lived in urban areas. The population is also characterized by its youth: 46.6% of the population is under 15 years of age. The vast majority of the Malian population is sedentary. Nomads represent 0.92% of the population and live mainly in rural areas .[28]

Mali comprises ten administrative regions (Kayes, Koulikoro, Sikasso, Ségou, Mopti, Timbuktu, Gao, Kidal, Taoudenit, Ménaka), 49 cercles, the district of Bamako (the capital) and 703 communes. The latter are administered by local authorities.

The Kayes region is Mali's first administrative region. Its regional capital is the town of Kayes. It is bordered to the south by Guinea, to the east by the Koulikoro region, to the north by Mauritania and to the west by Senegal .[29]

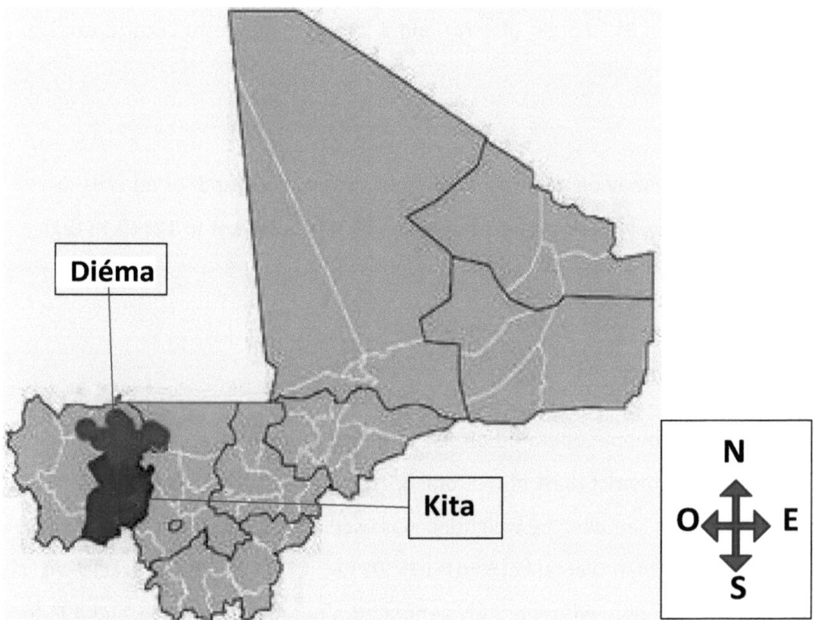

Figure 2: *Health maps of Kita and Diéma*[30]

Our study was carried out in the health districts of Kita and Diéma in the Kayes region of Mali. These two districts were chosen because, during the study period, they were the only ones to perform trichiasis operations in the HKI intervention zone.

1.2. Type of study:

This was a descriptive cross-sectional study.

1.3. Study population :

All patients operated on for trachomatous trichiasis in the Kita and Diéma districts during the period from January 1er to December 31 2017.

1.4. Sampling :

The sample size was calculated with Epi info7 software, using Statcalc with a 95%

confidence interval, an 8% margin of error and a 28% prevalence of recurrence[bl2] i.e. 121 participants.

(N = 121 individuals).

Considering that there may be non-respondents (absent or deceased) or refusals to participate in the study, we calculated a margin of 10%, equivalent to 121+0.1 (121). =121+12=133

For all participants, the method was probabilistic.

Sampling technique :

Out of a total of 492 people operated on for TT in the Kayes region in 2017, including 403 in the Kita health district (82% of the total operated on) and 89 in the Diéma health district (18%), random sampling by weighting was used. This gave us n1=133*0.82=109 in Kita; n2=133*0.18=24 in Diéma, i.e. N=n1+n2=109+24=133. Then, using Excel's "ALEA between Bounds" function, we separately generated a number between 1 and 403 for the Kita health district and from 1 to 89 for the Diéma district, in order to randomly select the 109 patients from Kita and the 24 patients from Diéma.

This sampling was carried out using the TT surgery database held by the PNSO and HKI.

1.5. Inclusion criteria:

Any person residing in the districts of Kita and Diéma without distinction who had undergone surgery for trachomatous trichiasis (TT) during the study period and whose verbal free and informed consent had been obtained.

3

1.6. Exclusion criteria :

People who had undergone surgery but did not live in the Kita and Diéma districts were not included in the study.

---

[2] These results are based on reports from various post-surgery monitoring missions at 3 and 6 months after the TT surgeries, carried out jointly by PNSO, CSRef and HKI staff.

1.7. Replacement criteria :

Persons who were impossible to locate geographically due to incomplete or erroneous addresses, as well as deceased persons, were replaced with the 10% margin.

1.8. Procedure :

Once our study protocol had been drawn up, it was submitted to and validated by the HKI coordination team, then by the coordinator of Mali's national eye health program (PNSO). Three teams of four people carried out the survey, including two teams in the Kita district and one in the Diéma district.

Before leaving for the field, we held a training and standardization session at the HKI office.

All teams had at their disposal a 4x4 vehicle with fuel, a cell phone and communication units to call participants the day before in preparation for the next day's meeting.

The study was funded by HKI bureau du Mali through its Projet d'Elimination du Trachome and covered the period from June 22 to July 1er 2017. Collection lasted ten days in Kita and five days in Diéma.

1.9. Benefits and risks of the study :

- **Study risks:** risks were minimized by disinfecting examiners' hands before each examination and wearing protective gloves during high-risk examinations.
- **The benefits of the study:** cases of recurrence or complications found were referred to be managed by a special mission on their agreement and free of charge.

- Other eye infections were treated with 1% tetracycline ointment or referred to the nearest health center if necessary.

1.10. Team composition: the teams were composed as follows:

- a Medical Assistant in Ophthalmology from the PNSO was in charge of examining the eyes. He had at his disposal: magnifying glasses providing 2.5 magnification (dioptres); a flashlight, disinfectant solution, 1% tetracycline ointments and reference cards.

- Participants were examined in their homes or in a shaded area, as intense sunlight produces shadows that make it difficult to observe the eyelid margin.
- The examination took place as follows: the examiner asked the patient to look straight ahead with eyes normally open. Using a powerful electric lamp, he illuminates the edge of the eyelid from below. He then looks upwards at the eyelid. He examines the rim where the eyelashes are implanted. Continuing to look down and sideways, he looks for downward-pointing eyelashes, to see if any are clearly touching the eyeball. He provided care when needed, and referred patients whenever necessary.

An interviewer who understood the local language and customs administered the questionnaire on a smartphone using the "ONA" application on the Open Data Kit platform.

We were among those who administered the questionnaire in a team.

The questionnaire consisted of 46 questions (see appended form) and was completed at the same time as the participants' eyes were examined. If the same patient had undergone several operations for trichiasis, the evaluation was based exclusively on the result obtained from the last eyelid operated on during the study period.

Administering the questionnaire took around 20 minutes, and all four eyelids and eyeballs were examined.

Information was collected directly on smartphones from each of the 125 participants included in the study.

- a "relay/community guide" was chosen locally for his knowledge of the locality, and above all for his regular contact with the people included in the study who live in his area. His task was to identify the homes of randomly selected people and make contact with them from the day before the survey. He accompanied the team throughout the process.

➢ a district ophthalmologist supervisor who was not one of those who had operated.

1.11. Parameters studied:

➢ **General information:** age, gender, eye operated on

➢ **The quality of the surgery***:* this was measured by assessing the functional status of the eye whose eyelid had been operated on, and whether or not there was any tearing, discomfort or itching in the eye.

➢ **Signs of recurrence:** i.e. depilation or signs of depilation and/or eyelash regrowth (especially in the median part of the free edge opposite the cornea), the existence of stitches.

➢ **Frequency of post-surgical complications:**

The existence of granuloma[c4] , drooping of the eyelid which closes the eyeball and requires overcorrection or even total non-closure of the eyeball at rest when closing the eyes, but also keloids at the suture point. An examination for eyelid occlusion defects was also carried out to see if the palpebral slit was not closing properly.

➢ **Information about the operation:** location of the operation, post-surgery medication, recommendations or instructions given after the operation.

➢ **Adherence to preferred post-operative care practices:** time for bandage removal, place of removal, who removed the bandage, time for suture removal, place of suture removal, who removed the suture, post-operative care received.

➢ **Patient satisfaction:** The **Likert Scale**[d5] was used to assess the degree of satisfaction of patients undergoing surgery.

In our context, it was: "Your vision has improved after eye surgery.
You are satisfied with the health of your eye following the operation" and "You are satisfied with the health of your eye following the operation" you are :

Totally disagree, Disagree,

---

[4] The term granuloma refers to a benign tumor of an inflammatory nature, consisting of connective tissue particularly rich in vessels, and penetrated by cells of various kinds. It may arise after TT surgery, and is not specific to any particular disease.

[5] A Likert scale is an attitude scale comprising 3 to 7 degrees in which the individual is asked to express his or her degree of agreement or disagreement with a statement.

No opinion, Agreed,

I couldn't agree more.[31]

1.12. Quality control :

To guarantee the quality of the results, we briefed the various team members on the collection tools, and a pre-survey was carried out after the training on 5 people not included in our sample, in order to test the collection tools.

The data, once entered on Smartphones, were recorded and sent to the PNSO's ODK platform account, after two stages of verification (the first by the interviewers themselves, the second by the supervisor, who is the project monitoring and evaluation manager at HKI).

1.13. Data analysis :

After verification, the data were transported and analyzed using EPI-INFO 7 and Microsoft Excel. For this analysis, we were supported by our internship supervisor and HKI Mali's follow-up evaluator.

Recurrence frequencies, percentage proportions and 95% confidence intervals were calculated. These consisted essentially of an analysis of the characteristics of those presenting with a recurrence, as well as an analysis of the frequency of complications and of the answers given by the patients who completed the questionnaire.

1.14. Ethical considerations :

This study is an ideal way of optimizing the quality of trichiasis surgery. It falls mainly within the scope of the PNSO's activities, and will therefore be beneficial rather than aggressive. As the PNSO was involved throughout the study process, the protocol was not submitted to the ethics committee.

The authorization of district administrative and health managers, as well as community leaders, was always sought. Confidentiality and, above all, respect for participants were respected.

True, this study was not invasive for the participants. However, an intervention proposal for patients with recurrences was made, and by an experienced ophthalmologist.

All study procedures were clearly explained to participants to ensure that they fully understood the purpose of the study and to obtain their free, informed, individual and verbal consent. Participants' rights and well-being were protected, and it was emphasized that the quality of their medical care would not be affected if they refused to take part in the study.

Study participants' names and personal information will remain confidential. The study will provide information to improve the quality of TT surgery. This information will be used by the PNSO to develop targeted interventions to improve the quality of TT surgery, with the ultimate goal of eliminating trachoma. Participants received no monetary compensation, however, their participation was highly appreciated and welcomed.

Free and informed verbal consent :

In order to take part in the study, the objectives of the survey were clearly explained to each eligible person. Verbal informed consent to participate was then sought, although the conduct of this type of study (observational in essence) presented no risk to the participant, nor raised any ethical issues. All those contacted were very happy to take part, and expressed their gratitude for the fact that they were treated at home, and for the fact that they could come back a year later to see how the operation had gone, all free of charge.

2. Results :

2.1. Recurrence and complications

Table 1: Characteristics of study participants (N=125)

Features		**workforce**	
		N=125	**%**
Districts	Kita	103	82
	Diéma	22	18
Gender	Female	77	62
	Male	48	38
Age range in years	35-45	11	9
	46-60	32	25
	61 and over	82	66
Number of eyelid operations per person		(n=167**)	%
	Right	41	32.8
	Left	42	33,6
	Both	84*	33,6
Number of operated eyelids with recurrence	Recurrence	25	14,9
Number of recurrences by sex		(n=25)	
	female	18	72
	male	7	28
Granuloma	yes	3	2
	no	122	98

**42 people had both eyelids operated on (42*2=84)*
***41 eyelids on the left, 42 on the right and 42 people for both eyelids, i.e. (42*2=84), making a total of (41+42+84=167) eyelids operated on.*

Of the 133 people, 8 did not participate in our study: (3 deceased; 4 not found due to inaccurate addresses or incorrect transcription of names; 1 case of displacement from his usual residence and outside the district). A total of 125 trichiasis patients took part in the study; 62% were female (95% CI [52.5% - 70.2%]) and 66% were over 60 (95% CI [57.4% - 70.2%]).

74,6%].

Examination of the operated eyelids revealed around 15% recurrence (at least one or more eyelashes directed towards the cornea, or presence of signs of epilation) at one year after surgery. Recurrence rates were higher in women (72%).

Only 3/167 cases, i.e. around 2%, were found to have granulomas.

Table 2: Information on TT surgery (N=125)

Intervention information	**workforce**		
		n	**%**
place of intervention	Patient's home	110	88
	Health center	15	12
Place of dressing removal	Patient's home	108	86
	Health center	17	14
Dressing removal time (*after surgery*) **(N=110)**[e6]	One day	70	64
	Two to three days	40	36
Person who removed the dressing	TT surgeon	88	70
	Other health agent	6	5
	Community Relay	19	15
	Family member	12	10
Suture removal t i m e (number of days) (N=91)	< 7	19	21
	≥ 7 days	72	79
Person who removes the wire suture	TT surgeon	97	77
	Other[f7]	28	23

In 88% of cases, TT operations were performed at the beneficiaries' homes, and suture removal was carried out by the surgeon in 77% of cases.

[6] Of the patients, 110 answered the question concerning the time taken to remove the dressing, which was 24 hours after the operation, as recommended by the WHO.

[7] thread that does not necessarily require removal can disintegrate or be absorbed over time, of which there are 7, and by another health agent, of which there are 21.

Table 3: immediate post-surgery medication.

Immediate post-op medication		Numbers (N=125)	
		n	%
Azithromicin tablet 250mg	Yes	83	66,4
	No	38	30,4
	Can't remember	4	3,2
Paracetamol tablet 500 mg	Yes	106	85
	No	16	13
	Can't remember	3	2
Tetracycline 1% ointment	Yes	121	97
	No	4	3

Immediately after the operation, 66.4% of those operated on had received azithromicin tablet 250 mg, 85% paracetamol tablet 500 mg, 97% 1% tetracycline ointment.

Table 4: Summary of instructions given after surgery.

Post-operative instructions		Numbers N=125	
		n	%
Instructions received	Yes		11995
	No	6	5
Information on taking medication	Yes		9681
	No		2319
Instructions not to touch the dressing	Yes		6353
	No		5647
Information on the surgeon's return for the removal of the bandage	Yes		8269
	No		3731
Information on the surgeon's return for suture removal	Yes		6655
	No		5345

Among the 95% who had received instructions after surgery, 81% were informed about taking medication, 53% knew that touching the operated eye could have consequences, 69% about the time required to remove the dressing, and 55% about removing the sutures.

Table 5: Impact of illness on quality of life

Difficulty performing daily tasks		Absolute frequency (N=125)	
		n	%
before the operation	Yes	109	87
	No	16	13
After the operation	Improved	118	94
	No change	7	6

More than half the people interviewed 87%, 95% CI [80.0% - 92.5%] stated that the disease prevented them from performing daily tasks with ease. After their TT operation, 94% confirmed that they were able to resume their daily activities without any problems 95% CI [81.9% - 93.7%].

Table 6: Vision status, evolution of signs and symptoms after surgery (N=125)

Absolute frequency (N=125)		
Feeling information	**n**	**%**
Improved vision	118	94
No improvement in vision	1	1
Indifferent	5	4
Blindness before surgery	1	1
Partial or total absence of signs/symptoms		
Yes	92	74
No	33	26

Although no visual acuity tests were carried out either before or after the operation, 94% of people stated that their vision had improved after the TT procedure. As for the partial or total disappearance of the signs and symptoms of the disease, 74% of individuals no longer complained of any symptoms.

Table 7: Frequency of signs and symptoms experienced before surgery by participants (N=125).

Signs/symptoms before surgery		Absolute frequency (N=125)	
		n	%
Pain	Yes	65	52
	No	60	48
Tearing	Yes	66	53
	No	59	47
Eye redness	Yes	5	4
	No	120	96
Sensation of a foreign body in the eye	Yes	77	62
	No	48	38

Based on how patients felt before the TT operation on their eyelids, 65 (52%) of them confirmed that they had experienced pain in the eye and 77 (62%) a sensation of a foreign body in the eye (Trichiasis) due to the eyelashes rubbing against the cornea, 66 (53%) had tearing and only 5 (4%) complained of redness of the eyeball.

2.2. Patient satisfaction:

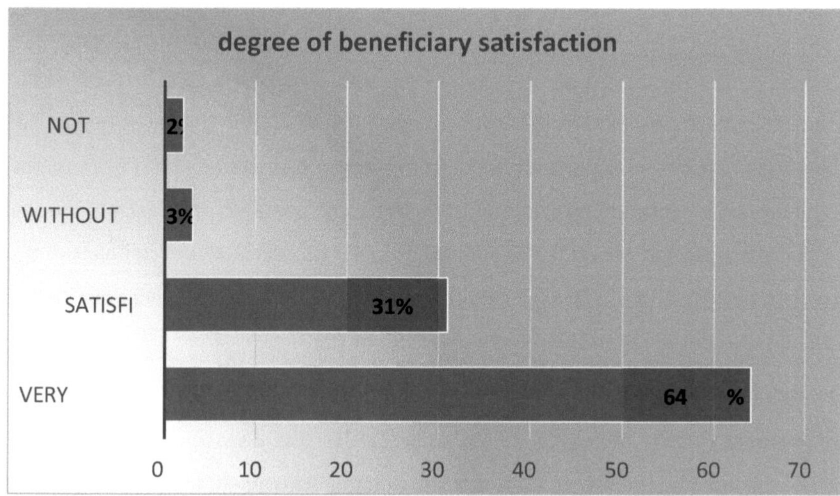

Figure 3: *Beneficiary satisfaction.*

95% CI agree [23.2% - 40.1%]; disagree [0.2% -5.7%] ;

Strongly agree [54.9% 72.4%].

For almost all patients questioned about their level of satisfaction with their vision or eye health, 64% were completely satisfied and said that TT surgery had improved their quality of life, and 31% were satisfied, for a total of 95% satisfied.

3. Discussion:

3.1. Socio-demographic characteristics:

Of the 133 patients sampled from the 492 operated on in 2017 in the Kayes region, 125 people took part in the study, with (82%) from the Kita district and (18%) from Diéma. This difference is explained by the proportion of people operated on in each of the said districts at the defined period. We would like to point out that HKI, which financed this study, is active in4 regions of Mali, including Kayes, in the fight against trachoma. Only in these two districts were interventions carried out in 2017.

The randomly selected sample was predominantly female (62%). This female predominance reflects the epidemiological forecast for the disease in Mali[32] . It could also be explained by the fact that children, in addition to women, are one of the most vulnerable groups to the disease. It should also be noted that once a mother and/or her child are infected, these mothers can reinfect themselves and their children if no hygiene measures are taken beforehand. The result is a lifelong cycle of infection. As a result, once these mothers reach an advanced age and develop complications from the disease, it's their children, and very generally their daughters, who in turn take care of them, hence the predominance of women. According to Schémann, in a study carried out in Mali in 2008, before the age of 20, active trachoma was still found in 13.5% of women. The prevalence then fell rapidly, to less than 3% over the age of 40. Conjunctival scarring (CS) was found in 27% of the women examined. Prevalence increased progressively with age, reaching 53.7% after the age of 70. The prevalence of entropion-trichiasis was 2.5% for all women in Mali. The frequency curve for entropion-trichiasis (ET) was similar to that for scarring trachoma, with the prevalence rate for trichiasis rising above the 1% threshold after the age of 30, reaching 10% after the age of 70[1] . Similar data were found by *Négrel et al in Morocco* in 2000 (63.8%)[33] , but this result is lower, than those found respectively by *Burton et al 2005* in Gambia (74.5%)[16] , and of (66.9%) by *Pearson K et al* 2013 in Ethiopia .[34]

More than half of the participants were over 60 years old (66%), with a median age of

65, with a minimum of 31 and a maximum of 101. These figures are higher than those found by *Pearson K et al* in Ethiopia with a median age of 49 in 2013[34] , as well as *Habtamu Esmael et al in Ethiopia 2016 (47 years)*[35] . They are similar to those of *Burton et al 2005 in Gambia* with a median age of 60 years and an interquartile range of 50 to 70 years[16] . This difference can be explained either by the rapidity of case management with the trachoma elimination campaigns in Ethiopia, or by the rapid progression to TT. It should also be remembered that around 70% of TT surgical cases are performed in Ethiopia.

3.2. Success and recurrence

Characteristics of operated eyelids on clinical examination:

All cases were operated on using the Trabut method, as this is the only technique practiced by TT surgeons in Mali.

Examination of the operated eyelids found 15% cases of relapse one year after surgery with a female predominance of (72%), which is superimposable on the 15.8% overall recurrence of *Négrel AD et al in Morocco in 1998* from 6 months after surgery, of whom 91.2% were operated on using the bilamellar tarsal rotation method (RBLT)[33] , but it is well below those found by *Khandekar R in Oman 2001* in an experimental study with 56% of all surgical cases recurring, of whom 50.6% of patients with electroepilation and 61.8% of patients with tarsal rotation[23] *. In the Gambia, Burton MJ et al* found 41.3% recurrence in 2011 in a cohort study on the long-term results of trichiasis surgery[16] *, West ES et al 2005,* reported 28% in an observational cohort study to investigate risk factors for trichiasis recurrence at 18 months post-surgery in a trachoma-endemic area of Tanzania, This study showed that time after surgery was not a risk factor for recurrence[36] , but that the frequency of recurrence was significantly higher than in our study. In the same vein, *Reacher MH et al Chicago1992 found* a 20% recurrence rate in a controlled trial of upper eyelid trachomatous trichiasis surgery in Oman (by tarsal rotation), which is higher than the results of our study, but at a follow-up of 9 and 21 months after surgery on 384 eyelids[37] . Fifty-six eyes showed recurrence at one year with an adjusted prevalence of (8.8%) and one hundred and one eyes (15.9%) recurred two years after surgery with the female gender incriminated by *Khandekar R et al* in the study of determinants of trichiasis recurrence, differing at one and two years after eyelid surgery in Vietnam[38] , these figures are comparable to those demonstrated in our study.

The study found that in 64% of cases, the one-day deadline for dressing removal was met in line with WHO recommendations, reflecting in part the degree of compliance with protocol in TT surgery .[39]

The study showed that suture removal was carried out at the patient's home in 73% of cases, with 74% within the recommended timeframe of 7 days after the TT surgeries (8ème days), as recommended by the WHO .[39]

We note that for almost all cases, surgery improved quality of life, even in cases of recurrence, as *Palmer SL et al* also demonstrated *in 2014* during a study on the qualitative assessment of quality of life in women with trichiasis in rural areas of Niger[40] .In the same study, all twenty-three women interviewed spoke of trichiasis as a "living death" because it causes intense pain, which affects quality of life with an inability to perform daily tasks, social events making it difficult to live in the community which is not without consequence on economic income in Niger.

Systematic treatment received immediately after surgery:

Immediately after surgery, 66.4% of those operated on had received the WHO-recommended azithromicin[39] . Other studies have shown the benefits of azithromicin in reducing the risk of recurrence, according to *Zhang H et al* in a *2006* randomized study of the impact of oral azithromicin on the recurrence of trachomatous trichiasis in Nepal over the course of a year and even at six months post-surgery, which found that recurrence was 28.9% at 12 months. This study also demonstrated that recurrence was significantly lower in patients with major TT at baseline in the azithromycin group at 12 months[41] . It was 10% in the azithromycin group and 13% in the tetracycline group according to a randomized, single-mask clinical trial conducted in southern Ethiopia, a region where trachoma is hyperendemic by *Woreta F et* al[42] . The Azithromycin-treated group showed a 22% reduction in trichiasis recurrence three years after surgery, compared with the tetracycline-treated group.This was not the case according to *Burton MJ et al*, who in a randomized controlled trial of Azithromycin after surgery for trachomatous trichiasis in The Gambia found that there was no difference in trichiasis recurrence between the Azithromycin group and the control group[43] . Many studies have been carried out on the postoperative outcome of TT surgery, but few of them have reported on the outcome of raking campaigns. This was also the context of this study.

Signs and symptoms before and after surgery:

Although no visual acuity tests were carried out either before or after the operation based on self-reporting, 94.4% of people reported improved vision after the TT eyelid procedure. These results are similar to those demonstrated by *Woreta TA et al* 2009 in Ethiopia in a study on the effect of trichiasis surgery on visual acuity .[44]

As for the complete disappearance of signs and symptoms of the disease and the improvement in quality of life after TT surgery, 74% of the individuals surveyed no longer complained of any symptoms.

Based on how patients felt before TT's eyelid surgery, 52% of them confirmed that they had experienced pain in the eye, 62% that they had felt a foreign body in the eye due to the eyelashes rubbing against the cornea, 53% that they had tearing and only 4% that they had complained of redness of the eyeball.

According to 74% of those who underwent surgery, the signs or symptoms of TT partially or completely disappeared after the operation, as opposed to 26.4% who experienced some minor signs at times (watering eyes) with considerable improvement. These results are similar to those found by *Burton MJ et al in Gambia in 2005,* where visual acuity and symptoms improved considerably after surgery[43] . The absence or reduction of signs or symptoms after surgery constitutes an improvement in quality of life even in the event of failure *Palmer SL et* al in Niger in 2014 .[40]

3.3. Types of complications:

With only 3 cases (2.4%) of granuloma reported in the study, we believe that TT surgery using the Trabut method is of acceptable quality and that in this case the results are encouraging, in contrast to those found by *Négrel AD et al in Morocco in 2000* with a complication rate of 9.7%[33] and granuloma formation were recorded in 10.5% by Gower et al in the study on the rate and risk factors of unfavorable outcomes 6 weeks after Trichiasis surgery[22] . The frequency of granuloma found by our study is much lower than the 0.6% granuloma rate of *Pearson K et al in Ethiopia*, who found other complications such as, eyelid closure defects 5.5% (95% CI: 3.4-8.4) and lid notching 16.8% (95% CI
13,1-21,1) .[34]

3.4. Patient satisfaction:

For almost all patients questioned about their degree of satisfaction with their vision or eye health, 64% were very satisfied with TT surgery, which they felt improved their quality of life. This is lower than the 86% very satisfied reported by *Oktavec K C. et al in Oman in 2015*[45] ,also 31.2% satisfied, giving a total of 95.2% satisfaction. Subsequently, (Pearson K and in Ethiopia in 2013), in a study evaluating community-based trichiasis surgery gives that the majority of participants reported being satisfied with the trichiasis treatment they had undergone[34] . Our frequency of overall satisfaction is higher than that of Bowman RJC et al with surgery (88%) in Gambia in 2000 after 10 years of follow-up .[46]

Limits and difficulties:

The aim was to study the quality of trichiasis surgery in the districts of Kita and Diéma in the Kayes region of Mali, and to assess the recurrence rate, frequency of complications and degree of satisfaction of patients operated on in 2017, i.e. 12 months after surgery. This study was the culmination of several post-surgery monitoring missions carried out by the PNSO with the support of HKI, which took place between 3 and 6 months after surgery, with a small sample and by health area, and which have never been published.

As with all human endeavors, our study has its limitations, including sample size. Since researching beneficiaries is logistically and time-consuming, we were obliged to increase the margin of error in order to reduce thesample size.

But also memory bias, given the age of the participants and the time elapsed between the operation and the study. The short duration of the course, and the logistical and financial resources available, meant that we couldn't do any better. It should also be noted that although the individuals selected at random all agreed to take part in the study after giving verbal informed consent, 8 of them could not be found for various reasons: 03 died, 05 could not be found because of incorrect addresses. The participants were all very happy with the fact that they had been operated on at home, at no cost to them, and then to come back a year later and see how they were doing was a first for them. And despite the difficulties involved, since it was also a question of finding the selected people in the villages where they lived, very often in the hamlets and during the winter months. On the other hand, the distance separating these homes, very often within a radius of 05 to 35 km from the health center, did not prevent us from obtaining results that we consider to be of good quality and very reliable.

The 20 surgeons who performed these TT surgical procedures were all certified for TT surgery according to the WHO certification method. However, it was very difficult to establish a link between the surgeons and the patients they operated on, as more than half (the patients) no longer knew where their TT surgery card was. And while the number of years of experience of the surgeons varied, from 4 to 20 years from the newest to the oldest, we have no idea how many cases were operated on per surgeon. Unquestionably, the most interesting experience is measured by the number of operations performed by each surgeon, so this is also one of the limitations of our study. Also, surgeons did not have personal registers in which they recorded the patients they operated on, which did not allow us to establish a link between them and their success rate. The absence of a database linking the surgeon to the patients he operated on was also a factor. Despite its limitations, the results of our study are comparable to those of other studies carried out elsewhere and can be implemented elsewhere.

NB: for the following reasons, some factors were not considered useful to study:

- The quality of the equipment and consumables used: because our study was carried out one year after the surgical procedure, we were unable to assess this aspect.
- Personal hygiene and the patient's living environment: the natural history of the disease shows that it is linked to insalubrity and a lack of individual and collective hygiene, as well as a lack of water. Once we were in the field, we realized that these same conditions were still present.
- Absence of a support person (patient companion) post-operation, often elderly people.
- Low economic income

Conclusion

Our study shows that TT surgery is of acceptable quality in these two districts of Mali's Kayes region, with a recurrence rate of 15%, and overall patient satisfaction of 95%. The fight against trachoma in Mali, through the implementation of the CHANCE strategy, is no longer far from the WHO's GET 2020 objective, but efforts remain to be made with regard to the factors associated with the very occurrence of trachoma (promiscuity, difficult access to water, hygiene, sanitation...). Given the importance of trichiasis surgery, regular, long-term follow-up is essential at this stage in the elimination of trachoma in Mali. There is no doubt that the fight against trachoma requires a synergy of action from all development players, as well as community involvement. While the commitment of governments and the strong mobilization of NGOs have not been lacking. Our visit to the area shows that there is still a lot to be done in terms of road infrastructure development and geographical and financial accessibility to healthcare. The patients we surveyed are still living in the same environment, so they remain exposed to trachoma. Until hygiene and sanitation measures are implemented, and trichiasis surgery projects - I was going to say, they must even precede surgery - I very much fear that we will be able to put an end to this scourge, which is ruining the quality of life of a population already disadvantaged by nature.

Suggestions :

Moreover, the impact of any poor-quality surgery can be profound. Given that repeat TT surgery is technically very difficult, given that a high proportion of recurrences will probably lead to an increase in cases of refusal of surgery by the community, which these days is not negligible in our country. We believe that..:

✓ that another study with more participants, on a larger scale and considering the factors linked to these recurrences in Mali, should be carried out at the end of the fight, given that the epidemiological recrudescence is possible.

✓ Reinforce post-surgery follow-up from 3 months or at most 6 months after the operation, in order to relieve patients in need as much as possible. This can also prevent or reduce the occurrence of certain complications, such as granulomas.

✓ Involve the communities concerned through village chiefs, women's organization representatives, teachers, community health workers, health extension workers or other front-line health workers.

✓ Recruit patients who are satisfied with their trichiasis operation to raise awareness of cases of refusal and encourage them to undergo surgery.

References:

1. Schémann J-F. Le trachome : Une maladie de la pauvreté. IRD éditions, 2008 http://books.openedition.org/irdeditions/2420.

2. Bickley RJ, Mkocha H, Munoz B, West S. Identifying Patient Peceived Barriers to Trichiasis Surgery in Kongwa District, Tanzania. *PLoS Negl Trop Dis 2017*; **11** :1-14.

3. Buchan JC, Limburg H, Burton MJ. Quality assurance in trichiasis surgery: a methodology. *Br J Ophthalmol* 2011; **95**: 331-334.

4. Taylor HR, Burton MJ, Haddad D, West S, Wright H. Trachoma. *The Lancet* 2014; **384**: 2142-2152.

5. World Health Organization. (WHO) Alliance for the Global Elimination of Trachoma by 2020. *Wkly Epidemiol Rec relevé Épidémiologique Hebd* 2018 ; **93** :371-80.

6. Moulin AM, Orfila J, Sacko D, Schémann J-F. La lutte contre le trachome en Afrique subsaharienne - *IRE Éditions* 2006 : 152

7. Palmer SL, Winskell K, Patterson AE et al. 'A living death'*:* a qualitative assessment of quality of life among women with trichiasis in rural Niger. *Int Health* 2014*;* **6**: 291-297.

8. WHO Priority eye diseases.

9. https://www.who.int/blindness/causes/priority/fr/index2.htl

10. World Health Organization. Trachoma. http://www.who.int/fr/news-room/fact-sheets/detail/trachoma.

11. Gambhir M, Basáñez MG et al. The development of an age-structured model for trachoma transmission dynamics, pathogenesis and control. *PLoS Negl Trop Dis* 2009 ; **3** : 462.

12. WHO. Trachoma elimination: accelerating action to reach the goal. www.trachomacoalition.org/sites/all/themes/report-2016/GET2020_2016_FR.pdf.

13. Bamani S, King JD, Dembele M *et al.* Where do we go from here? Prevalence of

trachoma three years after stopping mass distribution of antibiotics in the regions of Kayes and Koulikoro, Mali. *PLoS Negl Trop Dis 201 ;* **4** :734.

14. Schémann J-F, Sacko D, Banou A, Bamani S, Bore B, Coulibaly S. Cartographie du trachome au Mali : résultats d'une enquête nationale.1998 ; **76** :8.

15. World Health Organization Programme for the Prevention of Blindness and Planning for Global Elimination of Trachoma (GET). Geneva: WHO, 1997 http://apps.who.int/iris/handle/10665/66170.

16. Alemayehu W, Kello AB. Trichiasis surgery: a patient-centered approach. *Journal of community eye health*. 2015; **12** :14.

17. Burton MJ, Bowman RJC, Faal H et al. Long term outcome of trichiasis surgery in the Gambia. *Br J Ophthalmol* 2005 ; **89** :575-579.

18. West ES, Mkocha H, Munoz B, et al. Risk Factors for Postsurgical Trichiasis Recurrence in a Trachoma-Endemic Area. *Invest Ophthalmol Vis Sci* 2005 ; **46** :447-453.

19. International Coalition for Trachoma Control (ICTC). Psychological Support Guide related to trichiasis.2013 published online July.

20. Kuper H, Solomon AW, Buchan JC, Zondervan M, Mabey D, Foster A. Participatory evaluations of trachoma control programmes in eight countries. *Trop Med Int Health TM IH* 2005 ; **10** :764-772.

21. Kostopoulou O, Grzybowski A, Trompoukis C. Trichiasis in ancient times. *Clin Dermatol*
2016 ; **34** :521-523.

22. Reacher MH, Muñoz B, Alghassany A, Daar AS, Elbualy M, Taylor HR. A controlled trial of surgery for trachomatous trichiasis of the upper lid. *Arch Ophthalmol.* 1992; **110**: 667-674.

23. Gower EW, Merbs SL, Munoz BE, et al. Rates and Risk Factors for Unfavorable Outcomes 6 Weeks after Trichiasis Surgery. *Invest Ophthalmol*. 2011; **52**: 2704-2711.

24. Khandekar R, Mohammed AJ, Courtright P. Recurrence of trichiasis: a long-term follow- up study in the Sultanate of Oman. *Ophthalmic Epidemiol.* 2001; **8:** 155-161.

25. Wondu A, Amir BK. Trichiasis surgery: a patient-centered approach. *Community Eye Health Review.* 2015; **12**: 2.

26. Traoré L, Moulin AM, Orfelia. Chapter 8. When and how to operate for trichiasis: indications, quality, delegation, coverage rate, strategy? In: Schémann J-F, ed. Lutte contre le trachome en Afrique subsaharienne. *IRD Editions*. 2006: 81-87.

27. Khandekar R, Thanh TTK, Luong VQ. The determinants of trichiasis recurrence differ at one and two years following lid surgery in Vietnam: A community-based intervention study. *Oman J Ophthalmol*. 2009; 2: 119.

28. UNDP in Mali. UNDP. http://www.ml.undp.org/content/mali/fr/home.html

29. Demographic and Health Survey. (EDSM V). 2012; published online 2013.

30. Kayes region. Wikipedia 2018 published online May 1.https://fr/region from kayes.org.

31. Local government in Mali. Wikipedia .2019 published online February 14.

32. LIKERT scales or summed rankings methods. https://docplayer.fr/Echelles-de-likert-ou-methode summed rankings.html

33. Schémann J-F, West S. Chapter 7. How to identify individuals or communities at risk of trachoma and its blinding complications: the fight against trachoma in sub-Saharan Africa. *IRD Éditions*. 2006: 61-76.

34. Négrel AD, Chami-Khazraji Y, Arrache ML, Ottmani S, Mahjour J. Quality of trichiasis surgery in the Kingdom of Morocco. *Cahiers d'études et de recherches francophones Santé*. 2000; **10**:81-92.

35. Pearson K, Habte D, Zerihun M, et al. Evaluation of community-based trichiasis surgery in northwest ethiopia. *Ethiop J Health Sci* 2013; **23**: 10.

36. Habtamu E, Wondie T, Aweke S, et al. Impact of Trichiasis Surgery on Quality of Life: A Longitudinal Study in Ethiopia. *PLoS Negl Trop Dis*. 2016; **10**: 1-17.

37. West ES, Mkocha H, Munoz B, et al. Risk factors for postsurgical trichiasis recurrence in a trachoma-endemic area. Invest Ophthalmol Vis Sci 2005; **46**: 447-453.

38. Reacher MH, Muñoz B, Alghassany A, Daar AS, Elbualy M, Taylor HR. A Controlled

Trial of Surgery for Trachomatous Trichiasis of the Upper Lid. Arch Ophthalmol. 1992; **110**: 667-674.

39. Khandekar R, Thanh TTK, Luong VQ. The determinants of trichiasis recurrence differ at one and two years following lid surgery in Vietnam: A community-based intervention study. *Oman J Ophthalmol.* 2009; **2**: 119.

40. WHO/Department of Neglected Tropical Diseases. Trachomatous trichiasis surgery. http://www.who.int/trachoma/resources/fr.

41. Palmer SL, Winskell K, Patterson AE, et al. 'A living death': a qualitative assessment of quality of life among women with trichiasis in rural Niger. *Int Health*. 2014; **6**: 291-297.

42. Zhang H, Kandel RP, Atakari HK, Dean D. Impact of oral azithromycin on recurrence of trachomatous trichiasis in Nepal over 1 year. *Br J Ophthalmol.* 2006; **90**: 943-948.

43. Woreta F, Munoz B, Gower E, Alemayehu W, West SK. Three-year outcomes of the surgery for trichiasis, antibiotics to prevent recurrence trial. *Arch Ophthalmol.* 2012; **130**: 427-431.

44. Burton MJ, Kinteh F, Jallow O, et al. A randomised controlled trial of azithromycin following surgery for trachomatous trichiasis in the Gambia. *Br J Ophthalmol.* 2005; **89**: 1282-1288.

45. Woreta TA, Munoz BE, Gower EW, Alemayehu W, West SK. Effect of Trichiasis Surgery on Visual Acuity Outcomes in Ethiopia. *Arch Ophthalmol.* 2009; **127**: 1505-1510.

46. Oktavec KC, Cassard SD, Harding JC, et al. Patients' Perceptions of Trichiasis Surgery: Results from the Partnership for Rapid Elimination of Trachoma (PRET) Surgery Clinical Trial. *Ophthalmic Epidemiol.* 2015; **22**: 153-161.

47. Bowman RJC, Jatta B, Faal H, Bailey R, Foster A, Johnson GJ. Long-term follow-up of lid surgery for trichiasis in the Gambia: Surgical success and patient perceptions. *Eye.* 2000; **14:** 864-868.

48. Standard TT patient follow-up protocol - english.pdf. *https://hkw.sharepoint.com/sites/kellernet/programs/NTD/Library/Standars/TT/patient/follow-up/protocol*

Appendices :

Activities	May				June				July			
Proposal and validation of dissertation project												
Literature review												
Questionnaire design												
Identification and training of interviewers												
Data collection and entry												
Drafting the internship report												
Presentation of internship report after validation												
Data analysis and dissertation writing												

Figure 4: *Activity timeline (Gantt chart)*

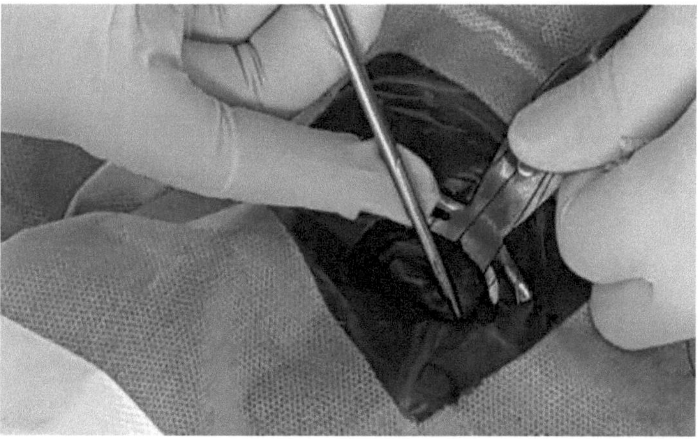

Figure 5: illustration *of trichiasis surgery using the Trabut method*

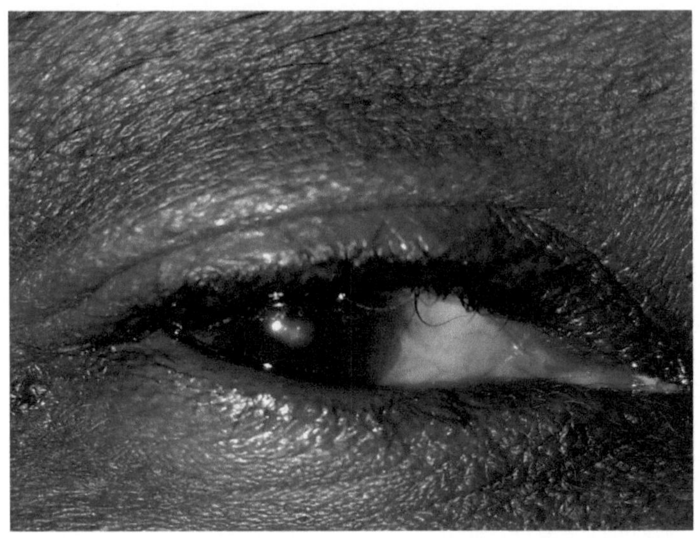

Figure 6: *illustration of a case of recurrent trichiasis with more than a few eyelashes directed towards the globe.*

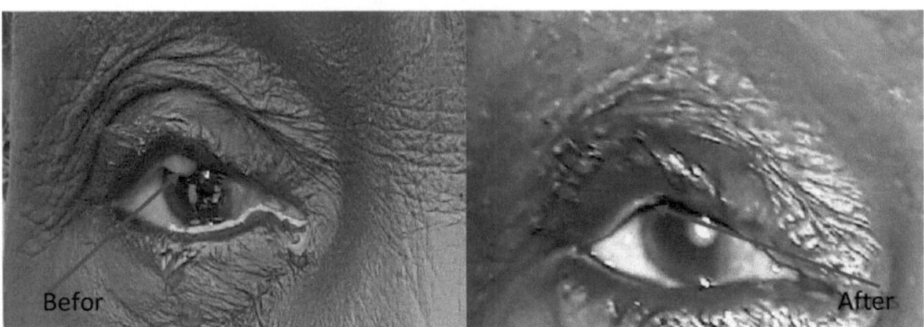

Figure 7: *A case of granuloma, in a 68-year-old woman at the time of the survey, excised by the ophthalmologist.*

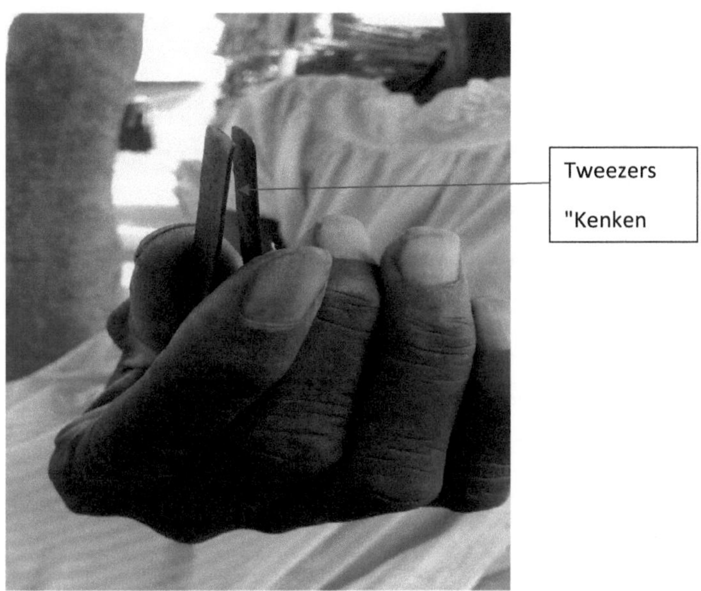

Figure 8: *An illustration of a pair of tweezers over 40 years old, with its owner, who has already undergone surgery, testifying to her satisfaction.*

TT post-operation follow-up data collection form

ID:/__/____/

Name of interviewer: /__________

Survey date:/____________/____/_/

I. General information :

1. District :________________

2. Health area ______________

3. Municipality______________

4. Village__________________

II. Patient information

5. Patient's first and last name _

6. Age in years : /_______/

7. Sex (M/F) :______________

8. Which eye did you have operated on?

OD☐ OG☐ ODG ☐

III. Clinical eye examination

➢ Right eye

Comments	YES	NO
9. does the patient have trichiasis on the operated eye?	☐	☐
10. The eyelid of the operated eye presents an abnorm	☐	☐
11. The operated eye shows a granuloma	☐	☐
12. The operated eye requires over-correction	☐	☐
13. The stitches are still in place	☐	☐
Other	☐	☐

Left eye :

Comments

	OUI	NON
does the patient have trichiasis on the operated eye?	☐	☐
The eyelid of the operated eye presents an abnormality	☐	☐
The operated eye shows a granuloma	☐	☐
The operated eye requires over-correction	☐	☐
Sutures are still in place	☐	☐
Other	☐	☐

IV. Intervention information :

14. Location where procedure was performed: health center:/_______ /at patients home:/_/

15. Date of intervention:/_______/____/____/

16. Eye operated for TT☐ 1.Right☐ 2.Left☐ 3.Both

17. Does the eye operated on correspond to the eye reported?☐ 1. Yes☐ 2. No

18. Who advised you to have the operation?________________________________

19. Did you receive any medication after the procedure? ☐ 1. yes☐ 2. No

20. If yes, which drugs? (show the patient the drugs and ask him to identify those he has received-DO NOT READ THE LIST BELOW)

21. Azythromycin ☐ 1. yes ☐ 2. No ☐ 3.don't know

22. Paracetamol ☐ 1. yes ☐ 2. No ☐ 3.don't know

23. Tetracyclin1% ointment ☐ 1. yes ☐ 2. No ☐ 3.don't know

V. Information on post-operative recommendations received

24. Did anyone give you any recommendations after the procedure? ☐1. yes☐2. no

25. If yes, what information did you receive? **(DO NOT READ TO PATIENT) :**

☐ Do not touch the operated eye

Instructions☐r taking any medication received

☐ Come back the next day to remove the bandage

☐ Come back in 7 days (after one week) to remove the sutures.

☐ Other :____________________

VI. Adherence to preferred post-operative care practices

26. How many days after the operation was the bandage removed?____________

Can' t remember ☐

27. Or has it been withdrawn?

☐ Hospital or health center☐ At home Other ______________________________

28. Who removed the bandage?

☐ Surgeon☐ social services☐ Family memberOther ______________

29. How many days after the operation were the sutures removed? ______________

Can't remember : ☐

30. Where were the wires removed? ________________________

☐ Hospital or health center☐ At home Other ______________________________

31. Who removed the sutures?

☐ Surgeon☐ social services☐ Family member Other________________________

32. Did you return to the health center for treatment of the operated eye (other than to remove the bandage or sutures):☐ 1. Yes☐ 2.No

33. If yes, why**? (DO NOT READ TO PATIENT)**

☐ General irritation of the operated eye☐ Excessive tearing

☐ Pain

☐ Other (associated with surgery - please specify)________________________

VII. Patient satisfaction :

34. Do you feel that your vision has changed since the operation?

☐ 1. yes☐ 2. no :☐ 3. indifferent☐ 4. not applicable (for people with a complete occlusion or blindness of the operated eye)

35. If so, how has it changed?

☐ 1. Improvement☐ 2.deterioration Other __________________________

36. Before surgery, did your trichiasis make it difficult for you to perform daily tasks?

☐ 1. yes ☐ 2.no ☐ 3. Don't know

37. Has your daily routine changed since your trichiasis operation?

☐ 1. Improvement ☐ 2.deterioration ☐ 3.no changeOther ____________

38. If improvement in what area?_

39. Was your eye painful before surgery? ☐ 1. yes ☐ 2.no

40. If yes, has the pain intensity changed since the procedure?

☐ 1. yes ☐ 2. no

41. If so, what changes?

42. ☐ 1. Improvement ☐ 2.deterioration Other ____________________

43. <<Your vision has improved after your eye surgery>>

☐ 1. Strongly disagree

☐ 2. Disagree

☐ 3. No opinion

☐ 4. I agree

☐ 5. Totally agree

44. Would you recommend surgery for trichiasis to someone with TT?

45. ☐ 1. yes ☐ 2. no : ☐ 3. indifferent

46. If not, why not?____________[47]

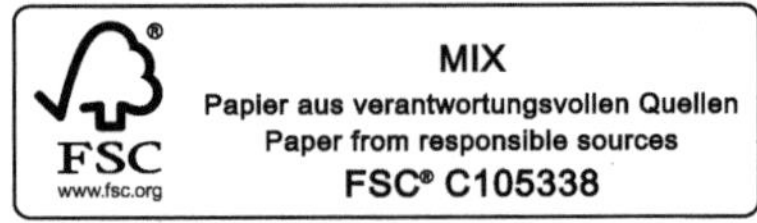

Printed by Books on Demand GmbH, Norderstedt / Germany